DMSO:

THE **MIRACLE HEALING** WONDER MEDICINE.

DMSO for Chronic & Other Related Diseases.

By

William Mattson.

Table of Contents.

SECTION A.

CHAPTER 1.

INTRODUCTION TO DIMETHYLSULFOXIDE.

As a Chemical, Pharmaceutical, and nutritional supplement is what best describes Dimethylsulfoxide (DMSO). It (DMSO) influences the body's proteins, carbohydrates, lipids, and water content while assisting medications in penetrating the skin.

Dimethylsulfoxide (DMSO), is a prescription drug that can be injected into the veins, administered topically, or consumed orally. It is an organosulphur compound with the formula C_2H_6OS.

It is also known to be a miracle medicine in most places around the globe, where it is predominantly used. This is because, it can be used to cure a variety of disorders in both people and animals, however, the FDA only advises using it on animals because of some negative effects that were noticed during the testing of the substance.

Numerous conditions, both slight and severe, have been treated with DMSO, including headaches, cancer, mental health issues, burns, interstitial cystitis, and many others. In this book, the uses and dosages of DMSO for each illness are spelled out.

The manufacture, usage, structure, and medical value of the dimethylsulfoxide (DMSO), are all thoroughly covered in this book. Students need to know this information for practical academic tests, and doctors need it for treating a variety of ailments.

CHAPTER 2.

DIMETHYLSULFOXIDE: WHAT IT IS.

It is an odorless liquid that disperses polar and non-polar substances and dissolves a variety of solvents, including H_2O (water). Thick rubber gloves are advised for handling DMSO because it easily penetrates the skin and has a flavor of oyster or garlic when it comes into contact with the mouth. DMSO is also known as methylsulfonylmethane, methylsulfoxide, and other names.

OBTAINING DMSO.

A Russian scientist named Alexander Saytzef created the substance for the first time in the middle of the eighteenth century.

DMSO is a by-product of wood pulp production; it is obtained during the production of wood pulp. In comparison to other substances of a similar nature, such as dimethylformamide, dimethylacetaldehyde, etc., DMSO may be a polar aprotic and less toxic.

Due to its great solvating power, DMSO is frequently employed for use as a solvent, primarily for chemical reactions involving nucleophilic reactions.

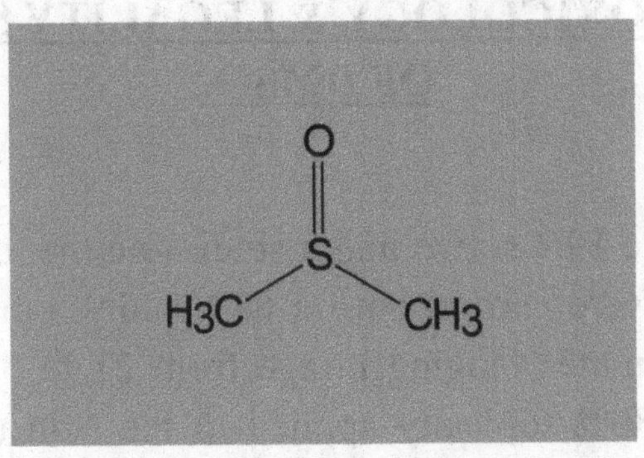

Below are some of the following characteristics of DMSO;

- ✓ 78.13grams per mol. in terms of molar mass.
- ✓ It has a high freezing point and is generally solid at room temp.
- ✓ It has no color.
- ✓ Its liquid density is 1.1004 g/cm3.
- ✓ *C_2H_6OS*'s molecular structure.
- ✓ The melting point is 18.5 °C (462K).

✓ Soluble in water, accompanied by a high boiling point.

CHAPTER 3.

THE TOXICOLOGY & LEGALITY STUDY OF DMSO.

In the late 1960s, two major studies on the toxicity of DMSO were carried out on 65 healthy, emotionally stable inmates ranging in age from 21 to 55. Using DMSO 80% topically applied to the skin at 1gram per kilogram of body weight per day for 14 days.

Only a small amount of skin scaling and drying returned to normal after a few days, some patients had lower systolic blood pressure, and all patients reported that DMSO had a taste that was comparable to garlic.

Although it is unknown if DMSO extends the life expectancy. However, given that it is a free radical scavenger and that radicals are helpful in the aging process, it may.

When high dosages of DMSO were given to certain animals in 1965, the lens of their eyes changed, however, this negative effect was reversed and the lens was restored to normal when therapy was stopped. Since the identical doses of DMSO did not cause these negative effects in either people or monkeys, the dimethylsulfoxide was declared safe for human usage.

THE LEGALITY OF DMSO.

According to research, Dimethylsulfoxide (DMSO) was licensed by the Food and Drug Administration (FDA) for use on horses, but some veterinarians also use it to treat laminitis and other inflammatory disorders.

All the above were before scientists conducted a study on it and discovered its medical usefulness, DMSO was initially utilized as an industrial solvent.

A short story was told of a woman who was treated in the early 1960s with sprained wrist with DMSO, it was said that she didn't get any better but instead, there were some noticeable more negative effects.

This gave a bad report on DMSO and it was greeted with misreactions from so many quarters.

Additionally, following some animal experiments, it was discovered that DMSO alters the refractive indicator of the lens in the eyes, leading to its ban but only approving it for a small number of uses, including organ preservation and the treatment of interstitial cystitis, a condition that affects the bladder.

The FDA authorized its use on animals (particularly horses and dogs) in the 1970s, in the routine treatment of inflammation and discomfort related to these animals.

The FDA approved the use of DMSO as a medication in 2007 to minimize brain-related problems that may emerge from traumatic injuries after structured medical hearings were held in this regard in the year 1980. Since then, DMSO has been used to treat a wide range of medical conditions.

Dimethylsulfoxide (DMSO) was licensed by the Food and Drug Administration (FDA) for use on horses, but some veterinarians use it illegally to treat other inflammatory conditions such as neurological issues and laminitis.

Before scientists conducted a study on it and discovered its medical usefulness, DMSO was initially utilized as an industrial solvent.

Early in the Eighteenth Century, studies commenced on the use of DMSO as a preservative for organs needed for transplantation began. Clinical trials on DMSO were discontinued in 1965 due to safety concerns, and it was only authorized for a limited number of uses, including organ preservation and the treatment of interstitial cystitis, a condition that affects the bladder.

SECTION B.

CHAPTER 4.

DIMETHYLSULFOXIDE'S CLINICAL BENEFITS AND HEALING.

Medical professionals utilize DMSO as a prescription drug and dietary supplement. It is one of the few substances that may be ingested through the mouth (oral ingestion), applied topically to the skin, administered intravenously through a vein, or injected into the body (whether as liquid, cream or gel).

When administered topically, the dimethylsulfoxide (DMSO) helps to ease pain and promotes a speedy recovery from burns, wounds, and other muscular problems.

The optimal DMSO texture for topical delivery is liquid or jelly-like. The ideal DMSO administration range is between 80% and 90%. The most typical way to apply DMSO is known to be topical administration.

In order to be administered orally, DMSO should not be taken in its 100% concentration alone. It needs to be used with other pharmaceutical ingredients in the ways that your doctor specifies or advises. It is advised to consume no more than two teaspoons daily.

The suggested dosage of administration shouldn't be greater than 50% for sensitive body areas like the face, neck, eyes, armpits, and others.

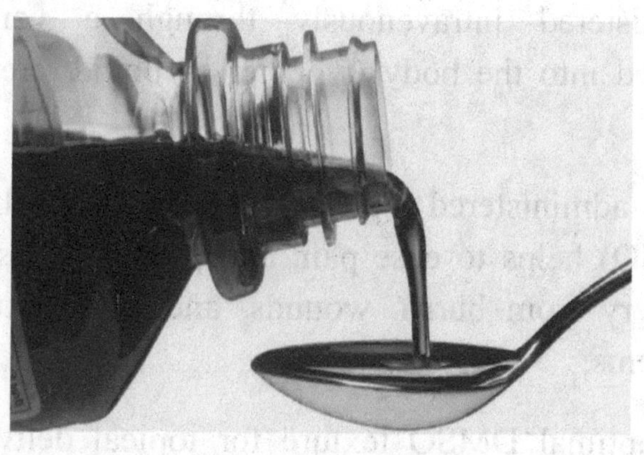

Following a series of studies, it was determined that DMSO has anti-inflammatory and health-promoting properties that make it an effective treatment for a number of debilitating conditions, including reflex sympathetic dystrophy, scleroderma, keloid scars, sclerosis, drug

extravasation injury, herpes, interstitial cystitis, and arthritis.

Bunions, toenail fungus, calluses, osteoarthritis, rheumatoid arthritis, intense facial discomfort (also known as tic douloureux), burns, bruises, and bruising are among the diseases it is used topically to treat.

In addition, it is utilized to treat problems of the eyes such as glaucoma, cataracts, and abnormalities of the retina. DMSO is used to treat bile stones and lower the abnormally high blood pressure in the brain in conjunction with other drugs.

DMSO is given topically to treat skin or tissue damage brought on by chemotherapy seeping through an IV during delivery.

<u>Nursing Mothers And Pregnant Women.</u>

Due to a lack of studies on DMSO in pregnant women, it should only be taken during pregnancy if the advantages outweigh the harm to the unborn child.

Because it makes some compounds more easily absorbed through organic tissues like the skin, DMSO is used as a medication delivery drug.

It dissolves compounds like organic salts, peptides, polymers, gases, and carbohydrates, it is often combined with oral medications to hasten absorption and improve its end results.

When given topically (5 grams per kilogram for 2 days, then 25 grams/kg for 10 days) and intraperitoneally (2 and ½ grams to 12 grams per day), DMSO produced teratogenic effects in animal tests. There were no issues with reproduction after oral/topical dosages.

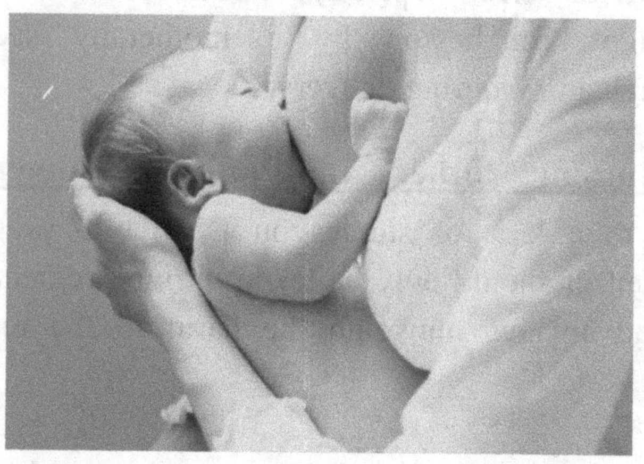

When giving DMSO to nursing women, it is suggested that care is needed due to the possibility of exposing newborns to medicines.

CHAPTER 5

THE USE OF DMSO TO TREAT AMYLOIDOSIS.

An uncommon condition called amyloidosis is brought about by the buildup of aberrant amyloid fibrils in tissues and organs, which alter their form and impair their function.

Protein polymers called amyloid fibrils exist. They are foreign materials that the immune system cannot readily identify or eliminate.

According to research, Men that are between the ages of 60-yrs and 70-yrs are more frequently affected by amyloidosis. Additionally, it can happen to dialysis patients with kidney dysfunction.

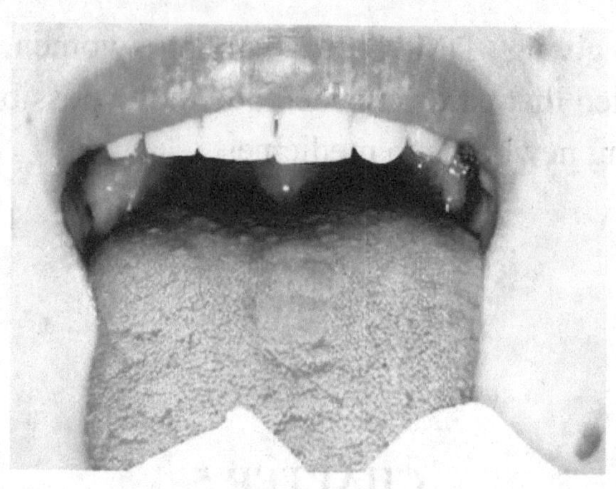

Symptoms and signs;

- ✓ Swelling of the ankles and legs,
- ✓ Shortness of breath with little effort,
- ✓ Extreme exhaustion and weakness,
- ✓ Numbness, pain, or tingling in the hands or feet.
- ✓ Loss of weight; diarrhea,
- ✓ An irregular heartbeat,
- ✓ Difficulty swallowing,

Additional forms of amyloidosis include;

> ➤ Primary amyloidosis (Primary AL) is another name for light chain amyloidosis (AL). It is the most prevalent form of amyloidosis in

industrialized nations, and it can damage nearly every organ, including the heart, kidneys, liver, peripheral nervous system, gastrointestinal tract, and respiratory tract. The bone marrow creates erratic antibodies when AL takes place.

➢ Amyloidosis (AA) with Inflammation: These conditions include rheumatoid arthritis, Crohn's disease, and ulcerative colitis. They are all chronic inflammatory diseases or systemic microbial infections. The kidney, liver, spleen, and heart are all impacted. It is also known as secondary Amyloidosis.

Other Amyloidosis include;
- ✓ Hereditary or familial amyloidosis,
- ✓ Wild Type Amyloidosis,
- ✓ Localized/Organ-Specific Amyloidosis,
- ✓ Dialysis-related amyloidosis.

The goal of treatment for amyloidosis is to control your symptoms while reducing the growth of the cycloid protein. DMSO is not a cure. According to a preliminary study, DMSO can be used to treat amyloidosis by applying it to the skin, using it to wash the bladder, or by ingesting it orally (mouth).

Amyloidosis is effectively treated by giving patients DMSO orally, typically for gastrointestinal and renal issues.

In a study involving some male and female humans that were between the ages of 23-yrs to 70-yrs, and who were diagnosed with secondary amyloidosis. But when they were orally treated with DMSO of 2g to 20grams per day, for about 7-wks to 8-weeks, there was found to be some good improvement.

CHAPTER 6.

DMSO AS A PAIN RELIEVER.

Pain can be managed topically using DMSO. Complex Regional Pain Syndrome Type 1, is the only painful disorder for which DMSO has been investigated in a number of controlled experiments, according to the research. The pain associated with CRPS 1 is a diverse syndrome defined by distributed pain, spreading edema, temperature abnormalities, and movement restriction after an initial detrimental event that progresses to pain unrelated to a typical injury.

Many pharmacological and non-pharmacological treatments for CRPS have not been supported by controlled research, but topical DMSO use has received some support for pain relief.

One clinical trial that randomly assigned 26 patients to receive either a regional intravenous sympathetic block or a 50% solution of DMSO provided evidence to support this result.

For three weeks, DMSO was applied four times each day. The daily activity and pain levels significantly improved.

Another study was discovered in the 2002 systematic review and judged to be of excellent quality. Thirty-two individuals were randomly assigned to receive 50% DMSO cream or a placebo cream in this randomized research.

After around two months, both groups exhibited significant reductions in pain and total symptom. Eleven patients additionally got physical therapy as the pain permitted.

In a random research with 146 patients, one group received one effervescent placebo tablet three times per day while the other administered 50% DMSO cream to the afflicted area five times per day.

A 600 milligram of N-acetylcysteine effervescent pill was administered three times daily to the second group, who also used a placebo cream five times per day. A free radical scavenger called N-acetylcysteine is used to treat Complicated Regional Pain Syndrome (CRPSI).

CHAPTER 7.

CARPAL TUNNEL SYNDROME DMSO APPLICATION AND RECIPE.

Carpal Tunnel Syndrome (CPS), is a chronic ailment that causes aches, numbness, itching, and overall weakness in the hands and wrists.

The median nerve, which supplies sensation to the index, thumb, middle, and half of the ring fingers, is under increased pressure in the wrist as a result of this condition.

Orthopedic surgeons have been aware of carpal tunnel syndrome for more than 30 years. Carpal tunnel syndrome surgery was initially performed in the early nineteenth century.

Symptoms include;
- ✓ Continuous wrist motion.
- ✓ Extreme wrist movements
- ✓ Vibration.
- ✓ Heredity.
- ✓ Pregnancy.

- ✓ Blood filtering (hemodialysis); • Dislocation and faction of the wrist; • Deformation of the hand or wrist; • Arthritis-related diseases; • Thyroid hormone imbalance.
- ✓ Diabetes
- ✓ Drinking too much alcohol
- ✓ A carpal tunnel tumor
- ✓ Finger tingling or discomfort (usually the thumb, index, and middle fingers).
- ✓ Weaker sensations at your fingertips.
- ✓ Trouble completing simple activities.
- ✓ Hand numbness or weakness.
- ✓ Dropping things.
- ✓ The inability to complete simple actions, like buttoning a shirt.

According to research, carpal tunnel syndrome pain can be reduced by applying DMSO 50% cream to the skin.

The therapy for carpal tunnel syndrome can be surgical or non-surgical; surgery is only done in severe situations. The non-surgical management of carpal tunnel syndrome includes DMSO.

CHAPTER 8.

FOR THE TREATMENT OF ATHLETIC INJURIES.

Athletes have used DMSO to treat injuries sustained during athletic competition, such as strains, sprains, bruises, and bone fractures, as well as to care for injured horses.

DMSO speeds up a repair, decreases pain and inflammation, and improves circulation. When used just after an injury, it functions more effectively.

Many athletes have seen the success of DMSO in curing injuries, despite the doubts of certain people, however, it functions differently for different people. Victims of serious injuries are encouraged to seek appropriate medical guidance before attempting self-healing.

However, administering DMSO as soon as the injury occurs can help prevent things from getting worse by halting the entire cycle of inflammation that signals the start of an injury.

Sports teams keep DMSO stocked near the sidelines for easy access to use on injured players right away.

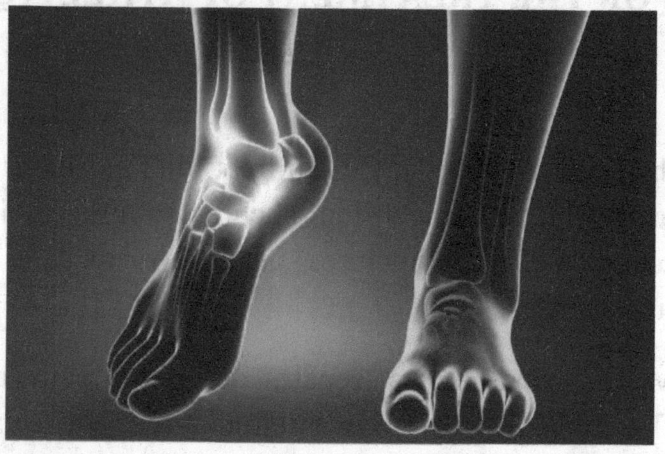

Applying 70% DMSO solution mixed with 30% peppermint oil topically or through spraying should be done every two to three hours for a period of seven to ten hours after the injury has been noticed, till a substantial improvement is noticed.

CHAPTER 9.

DMSO FOR THE TREATMENT OF DEMENTIA AND ALZHEIMER'S.

A neurodegenerative condition called Alzheimer's Disease (AD), causes the brain to shrink and the death of brain cells. In most cases, it typically begins slowly, gets worse over time, and progresses to dementia.

The disorder known as dementia is brought on by abnormal brain changes and has an impact on a person's ability to think, act, and interact socially. Microscopic bleeding, blood vessel blockages in the brain, and some treatable disorders including thyroid issues and vitamin shortages are other causes of dementia.

Studies show that millions of persons worldwide who are over the age of 65 and have dementia are believed to have Alzheimer's disease. In the United States, 5.8 million people with this disease have it, and of those 80% are over the age of 75-yrs.

The brain proteins beta-amyloid and tau, which are degenerating, are known to have an impact on the functionality of brain neurons, thereby causing damage, loss of connections, and death. The precise origin of Alzheimer's disease is unknown, but genetic changes can occasionally cause Alzheimer's disease.

Signs and symptoms;

Depending on the individual affected and the portion of the brain implicated, symptoms vary and the condition worsens in different ways. The majority of the time, it gets worse during times of stress, illness, or weariness.

- ✓ Forgetting familiar faces and locations.
- ✓ Difficulty understanding instructions and queries.
- ✓ A decline in social skills.
- ✓ Unpredictability in emotions.
- ✓ Consistent and frequent memory loss, especially of recent events.
- ✓ Poor clarity in daily communication.
- ✓ Decreased zeal for a formerly enjoyable activity.

Plaques and tangles eventually cover the entire brain, and the brain's tissue begins to shrink. In this severe condition, sufferers are fully dependent on others for their maintenance and are unable to communicate. As the body shuts down toward the end of life, the person might spend all of their time in bed.

Diagnosing Alzheimer.

Currently, there is no one test available to identify whether a patient has Alzheimer's disease. Only after thorough clinical consultation may the diagnosis be made.

The clinical diagnosis may consist of;

- ✓ A comprehensive physical and neurological examination.
- ✓ Tests on cerebral spinal fluid require lumbar puncture.
- ✓ Diagnostic imaging (whether MRI or PET).
- ✓ A complete medical history.
- ✓ A neuropsychological test, a psychological evaluation, an intellectual function test, and blood and urine testing.

DMSO has widespread use in clinical and preclinical studies as a vehicle for the entrance of water-insoluble drug candidates into the Central Nervous System (CNS).

It exhibits pharmacological effects and it performs beneficial biological activities due to its effects on the central nervous system, DMSO is important for the treatment of Alzheimer's disease and dementia.

It induces its effects on Alzheimer's both in-vitro and in-vivo species.

Treatment;

The amount and length of the treatment affect how effective DMSO is. The consequences of low dosages delivered in-vivo and in-vitro are difficult to determine, however, DMSO concentrations of 10% and above are hazardous in-vivo. The central nervous system is protected when DMSO is applied over a prolonged period.

CHAPTER 10.

ARTHRITIS TREATMENT WITH DMSO.

A rheumatic condition that affects one or more joints, the tissues surrounding the joints, or other connective tissues, arthritis is an inflammation of the joints. There are numerous different forms of arthritis, with rheumatoid arthritis and osteoarthritis being the most prevalent.

Children and adults of all ages can get arthritis, although individuals that are 65-yrs and older are more likely to develop it than adults of any other age group. Women tend to notice it more frequently than men do, and overweight persons are more likely to get affected.

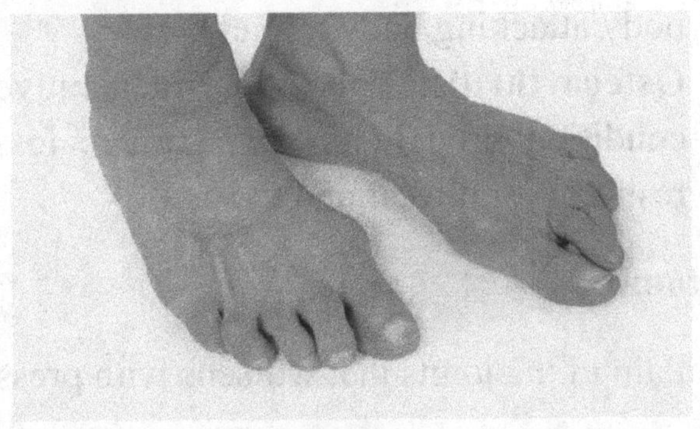

Symptoms;

- ✓ Reduced joint mobility, perhaps related to deformity.
- ✓ Skin nodules.
- ✓ Numbness, tingling, or burning feelings in the hands and feet.
- ✓ Problems falling asleep.
- ✓ Pleurisy-related chest pain when breathing in mouth and eyes are dry.
- ✓ Stiffness in the morning lasts for roughly an hour.
- ✓ Oftentimes, similar joints on both sides of the body experience pain.

- **Rheumatoid Arthritis:** Rheumatoid arthritis is brought about by the immune system of the body attacking body tissues.
- **Osteoarthritis:** This is a degenerative joint condition brought on by cartilage loss as a result of joint wear and tear.

Symptoms;

- ✓ Pain in the joints that worsens with pressure,

- ✓ A rubbing, grating, or crackling sound as the joints move,
- ✓ Pain-related sleep problems,
- ✓ Stiffness and pain in the joints.

Methylsulfonylmethane (MSM), which is found in green plants, fruits, and vegetables, and dimethyl sulfoxide (DMSO), both of which have similar pharmacological effects, are used to treat arthritis. They deduced from the research on osteoarthritis that MSM demonstrated restrained effectiveness; they did not assess DMSO. Methylsulfonylmethane (MSM) and Dimethylsulfoxide (DMSO) lessen arthritis, inflammation, and peripheral discomfort, and they may also prevent the degenerative effects of these conditions. Their sulfur concentration helps correct dietary sulfur deficits and enhance cartilage production.

DMSO can easily permeate the skin because it is a topical agent. When administered therapeutically, it is diluted.

<u>**Arthritis Treatment Recipe (Dosage):**</u>

To achieve a clinical effect, doctors urge osteoarthritis sufferers to utilize it for at least 3 months. As no dose-ranging studies are carried out, the ideal dosage for this DMSO in osteoarthritis has not been thoroughly studied.

Research has it that the therapeutic range for DMSO is 50% to 80%, while doses below 10% are considered clinically inactive.

CHAPTER 11.

DMSO RECIPE AND APPLICATION FOR DIABETES TREATMENT.

Diabetes is a condition that develops when the pancreas produces insufficient insulin or when the body cannot utilize the insulin that is produced effectively. This causes elevated blood sugar, or hyperglycemia, which over time negatively impacts the body systems, particularly the blood vessels and nerves, and causes serious damage.

■ Diabetes Type 1.

Previously, this was referred to as an insulin-dependent, juvenile, or childhood-onset condition as a result of inadequate insulin production. Although the reason and prevention actions are unknown, daily administration is necessary.

Excess urine is excreted, along with thirst, frequent hunger, weight loss, visual abnormalities, and exhaustion.

- ## <u>Diabetes Type 2.</u>

Previously, this was referred to as a non-insulin-dependent diabetic condition. It is brought on by the ineffective administration of insulin, being overweight, and not exercising enough.

The most common form of diabetes is this one. Both adults and children can get it.

- ## <u>Pregnancy-Related Diabetes.</u>

This is hyperglycemia, which is characterized by a high blood glucose level that is lower than that of people with diabetes. It happens throughout pregnancy.

Even after giving birth, problems remain a possibility for pregnant women with gestational diabetes.

There is a chance of difficulties during pregnancy and delivery for women with gestational diabetes. Future type 2 diabetes occurrence, is a danger for both these women and their offspring.

Diabetes over time can have an impact on the kidneys, nerves, blood vessels, heart, and eyes. Diabetes increases the risk of heart attacks in adults. Reduced blood flow, and nerve damage (neuropathy) in the feet increasing the risk of foot ulcers, infection, and even amputation of limbs are some complications of diabetes.

A good diet, frequent exercise, and blood sugar testing can all help with early diagnosis.

According to recent studies, DMSO has an immunomodulatory role and can thus be utilized to treat diabetic patients due to its diabetogenic action on the DNA and beta-cell membrane.

A two (2%) or three (3%) DMSO solution is useful for treating diabetes, according to prior experiments.

CHAPTER 12.

DMSO FOR BRAIN INJURY TREATMENT.

Worldwide, traumatic brain injuries rank as the leading cause of death. A strike or injury to the head that occurs as a result of physical activity, sports-related injuries, automobile accidents, military service, or acts of violence can cause traumatic brain injury.

Traumatic brain injuries affect everyone, regardless of age, profession, geography, or financial background. Millions of individuals are generally affected annually.

Males between the ages of 15-yrs and 24-yrs, adults, particularly women over the age of 65-yrs, and small children under the age of 4-yrs are more likely to experience it frequently.

After inducing traumatic brain injury in the mice, DMSO was injected intraperitoneally and continued to be given daily for the following seven days. DMSO was administered intraperitoneally or in vivo to mice for seven days at a dose of 5-milligram per kg per day. Humans may use this formula, but only under the guidance of your doctor's prescription.

CHAPTER 13.

DMSO AS A BURNS TREATMENT.

One of the most frequent, complicated, painful, and expensive physical injuries is burns. Burns are defined as first-degree (affecting the superficial sections of the epidermis), second-degree (either superficial or deep and affecting the entire epidermis), third-degree (loss of parts of the epidermis and dermis), and fourth-degree (including the loss of the entire epidermis, all the skin, the muscles below, bones and ligaments).

SSD (silver sulfadiazine) 1% cream is frequently used for the topical treatment of burns in humans and animals due to its antimicrobial efficacy due to its adverse side effects, it is best to look for another agent with lesser side effects. The treatment of burns in humans involved antimicrobial control of the infection due to the wound and analgesia.

DMSO is applied topically as an analgesic, a carrier for medications, an antioxidant, and an anti-inflammatory agent. Through its influence on cell

CHAPTER 14.

DMSO FOR THE TREATMENT OF HEARING AND EAR PROBLEMS.

Many individuals worldwide suffer from hearing loss, which can affect one or both ears and can range in severity from mild to severe. It often affects those that are over 60yrs of age, but it can affect people of all ages in general.

The following elements may contribute to hearing loss;

- ✓ When a person is older than 60.
- ✓ Constantly being around loud sounds.
- ✓ Having a family history of a genetic condition associated with hearing loss.
- ✓ Drugs that cause ototoxicity.

Head Injury: conditions such as autoimmune disease, otosclerosis, or Meniere's disease.

There are several different types of hearing loss, including:

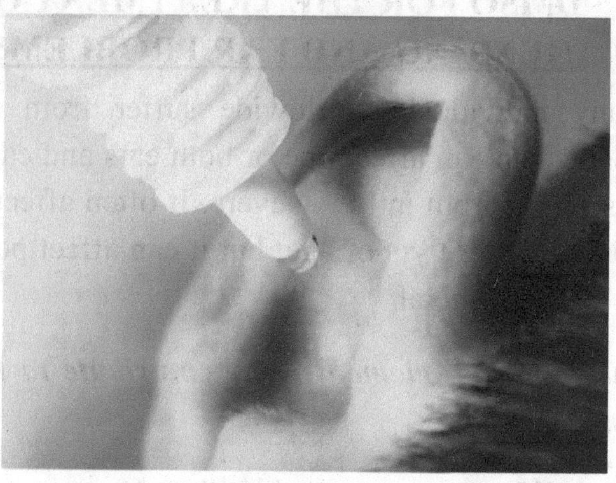

> **The Conductive hearing loss:** This is typically transient but might be permanent. It is brought on by a mechanical issue in the middle or outer ear or an obstruction in the ear canal.

> **Sensorineural hearing loss** is a permanent loss of hearing brought on by disorders that harm the microscopic hair-like cells in the inner ear (auditory nerve). Additionally, it makes it challenging to

comprehend speech and other sounds, even when they are quite loud.

Treatment Plan: Laboratory and clinical tests, including double-blind studies employing DMSO on patients with otological infections, revealed that applying a 90% DMSO had no antibacterial, anesthetic, anti-inflammatory, or ototoxic characteristics/effect when placed within the ear.

CHAPTER 15

RECIPE AND DMSO APPLICATION FOR THE TREATMENT OF EYE PROBLEMS.

Eye issues can be simple and go away on their own, and in other cases, serious and need an expert.

The most common types of eye issues include the following;

- ✓ Eyestrain,
- ✓ Red eyes,
- ✓ Night blindness,
- ✓ Lazy eyes (amblyopia),
- ✓ Crossed eyes (strabismus),
- ✓ Nystagmus,
- ✓ Color blindness,
- ✓ Uveitis,
- ✓ Presbyopia,
- ✓ Cataracts,
- ✓ Glaucoma,
- ✓ Retinal disorders,
- ✓ Conjunctivitis (Pinkeye),
- ✓ Corneal diseases,

- ✓ Eyelid issues, and changes in vision with age.

Retinitis Pigmentosa is the most frequent cause of blindness, and DMSO has been shown to be beneficial in treating it.

Fifty patients with macular degeneration were the subject of research that revealed some improvements. Improvements were noted after he administered 50% DMSO by eyecup twice daily for three months, to a patient with retinitis pigmentosa.

Many doctors have reported positive results after using an eyedropper to apply a 40% DMSO solution to the eye to treat the young and old for vision difficulties; after one week, patients were able to read the fine print.

Treatment of eye issues involves putting a drop of DMSO 25% solution in the eyes once or twice daily.

CHAPTER 16.

DMSO AS A HEADACHE TREATMENT.

Headaches are a fairly frequent ailment that people suffer from all around the world. They are characterized by persistent, throbbing pain that can lead to melancholy and anxiety. There are two types of headaches;

- ✓ The Primary Headache and
- ✓ The Secondary Headache.

While the secondary headache is caused by other medical problems such as head injury, hypertension, infections, trauma, tumors, and sinus congestion, the primary headache is not caused by any medical condition, such as migraines.

Children who get migraines typically inherit the condition from their parents because migraines have a strong propensity to run in families.

Additionally, household factors including ingesting caffeinated foods, alcohol, fermented foods, chocolate, cheese, and allergies might result in headaches.

In most cases, the interplay of impulses inside the brain, blood vessels, and nerve fibers causes headaches. Pain signals are conveyed to the brain by nerves that have been triggered by unidentified causes, resulting in headaches.

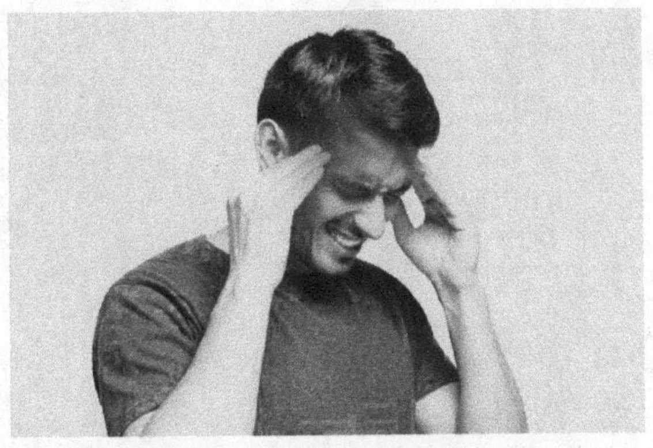

It is advised that you seek medical counsel or use DMSO if you frequently or severely have headaches.

Vascular headaches and muscular stress frequently coexist, and DMSO is an effective treatment for both. Use DMSO 90% solution on places with hair, such as your scalp or the areas around your temples. It can also be applied close to the eyes. DMSO does not always or always function, and this is true for both migraine.

CHAPTER 17

USING DMSO TO TREAT INFECTIONS & CYSTITIS.

You can take DMSO by itself or in conjunction with antibiotics. Bacteria that are resistant to an antibiotic become susceptible to that antibiotic when combined with DMSO. Clinical usage requires between 80% to 90% of DMSO. Additionally, DMSO can assist in delivering antibiotics to hard-to-reach body parts like the brain and bone marrow.

The virus's protein coat can be broken down by DMSO, exposing the virus's nucleic acid and core to the immune system. Additionally, it can be used topically to treat shingles-related lesions.

DMSO can quickly clear congested sinuses when applied topically to the face or nose. DMSO can also be applied topically on gum disease to lessen tooth pain and decay.

When used with 20mg of doxycycline, several individuals claim that using DMSO significantly reduced the severity of a mouth infection.

DMSO AS INTERSTITIAL CYSTITIS TREATMENT.

Interstitial cystitis is a bladder condition marked by pelvic pain, urgency during urination, and bladder pain.

Depending on the intensity, interstitial cystitis symptoms might linger for more than a month. The following signs are most frequently reported;

- ✓ Regular urination,
- ✓ Painful sex,
- ✓ A decrease in the volume of the bladder,
- ✓ And changes in sexual intimacy are all symptoms of chronic pelvic pain,
- ✓ As well as discomfort in the lower abdomen, back, and vagina.

For a speedier recovery, interstitial cystitis patients are advised to avoid certain foods, such as tea and coffee, soda, alcohol, citrus, cranberries, and nuts.

DMSO is a successful treatment for both of the two primary kinds of interstitial cystitis, viz-a-viz; ulcerative and non-ulcerative interstitial cystitis.

Interstitial cystitis-related edema and discomfort are lessened and the availability of blood to the treated areas is increased by DMSO.

A catheter device or tube is used to administer the DMSO 50% intravesical solution, which is then left in the bladder for up to 15 minutes or as prescribed by a doctor before being removed via urination. Patients are typically instructed to repeat this operation every two weeks until their symptoms are gone, but you should carefully follow your doctor's instructions.

It is not recommended to administer DMSO 50% intravesical solution via injection into a vein, muscle, or joint or to implant it in the bladder along with other drugs.

In order to facilitate the easy absorption of other medications infused into the bladder, such as heparin, steroids, bicarbonate, and analgesics, some healthcare providers add DMSO 50% to bladder cocktails. However, research has led to several changes regarding the medications mixed in bladder cocktails.

CHAPTER 18.

DMSO AND STANDARD THERAPY FOR PATIENTS WITH CANCER.

DMSO is useful for treating cancers like lymphoma, colon cancer, and melanoma as well as other types of cancer.

Two human intravenous DMSO cancer investigations, one on prostate cancer and the other on gallbladder cancer, were published by scientists. In these investigations, DMSO was infused intravenously five days a week together with baking soda (sodium bicarbonate). Clinical improvements in blood tests, quality of life, and symptoms were seen with few negative side effects.

You should use DMSO for six (6) weeks to eight (8) weeks to see if it will work to treat your cancer; for a slow-growing disease, a longer course of treatment is advised.

By converting quickly proliferating cells to normal ones and activating the tumor-suppressing protein. DMSO aids in the treatment of cancer by reducing the number of nearby malignant tumor cells and decreasing the progression of the disease.

DMSO has the power to stop the development of cancer cells. Patients are cautioned not to start any treatment without first seeking the counsel of a cancer-care specialist because more study has to be done in this area. At this time, additional research is still required to get a firm judgment regarding the effectiveness of DMSO in the treatment of cancer.

CHAPTER 19.

STROKE TREATMENT DMSO APPLICATION AND RECIPE.

When given as soon as a stroke occurs, DMSO dissolves the clot that causes it, restores circulation, and prevents paralysis. DMSO can be ingested, smeared on the skin, or administered intravenously (IV). It permeates the body and crosses the blood-brain barrier; while oral ingestion is effective, IV administration is advised.

Although DMSO-40% prolongs the bleeding period, it is still advised for usage in the management of embolic or hemorrhagic stroke. The best treatment for brain wounds, particularly in severe bleeding situations, is DMSO.

An intravenous solution of dimethylsulfoxide (DMSO of 560miligram per kilogram, 28% solution) and fructose 1,6-diphosphate (FDP: 200-miligram per kg, to be dissolved in 5% dextrose water solution) was administered twice daily for 12 days to assess the efficacy of DMSO in combination with FDP for the treatment of stroke. There was a noticeable improvement.

<u>USING DMSO TO TREAT GUM AND TOOTH DISEASES.</u>

Periodontal disease, which affects the supporting structures of the teeth, the periodontal membrane, the gums, and the bones and is brought about by poor oral hygiene, a diet deficient in nutrients and high in refined carbohydrates, is the leading cause of tooth loss in elderly and aged people.

DMSO is effective at preventing the growth of microorganisms and health problems.

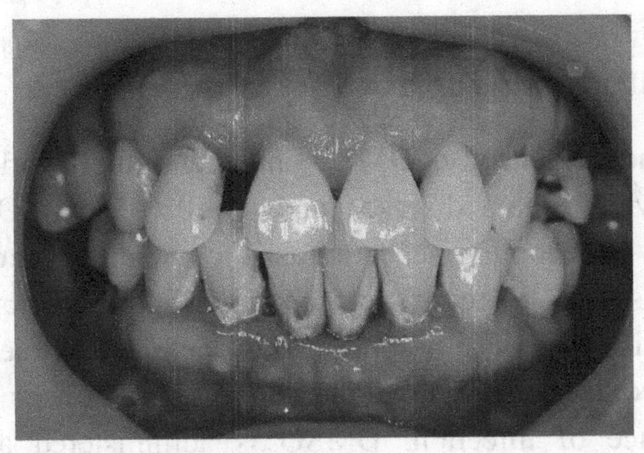

A study employing complex containers of 30% DMSO was done on fifty patients with periodontal disease. Of these, eighteen (18) had gum inflammation and bleeding, thirteen (13) had bleeding and swollen gums, and nineteen (19) had damaged periodontal disease that led to the loss of teeth and bone.

Patients in the early stages reported that some of the teeth tightened up and that the discomfort they typically felt decreased after receiving DMSO treatment. It was also discovered that patients treated with DMSO experienced less pain, bleeding, and inflammation. The improvement of disease-related foul breath was made possible by DMSO's capacity to kill microorganisms.

Some dentists use DMSO in their dental work to alleviate pain, disease, and swelling. DMSO is slowly becoming accepted as a medicinal treatment across the globe. It may be taken alongside other medications or antibiotics. After teeth are extracted, it works well to treat the gingiva and lowers the chance of infection. DMSO is administered after extractions to relieve toothache discomfort brought on by the procedure.

Many people use 50% DMSO as a mouthwash, while others only use it when they have a toothache to lessen the discomfort before visiting a dentist.

CHAPTER 20.

LAETRILE AND DMSO IN THE TREATMENT OF CANCER PATIENTS.

It was first used in the nineteenth century, and it is still used today to treat cancer when combined with laetrile. After the initial treatment, the patients continue to take laetrile pills and DMSO orally.

Other options for treatment include;

- ✓ Intramuscular injections,
- ✓ Topical applications directly to the malignancy,
- ✓ Intravenous injections via slow drip or push and,

✓ Intramuscular injections.

DMSO-laetrile intravenous combination was used to treat a woman with tongue cancer and staphylococcus infection on a second trial, and she made a full recovery. Nevertheless, she continued using DMSO and laetrile tablets for a while after her recovery to reduce the likelihood of cancer recurrence.

Laetrile and DMSO have been effectively used by many medical professionals from the USA, Mexico, and other nations to treat patients with terminal brain, liver, pancreatic, and other cancers. They claimed throughout their testimony that the procedure is less harmful than chemotherapy while yet being more effective.

<u>DMSO APPLICATION AND AWARD FOR LUPUS TREATMENT.</u>

The immune system is impacted by lupus, which causes it to assault body tissue and cause harm.

Depending on the individual, some of the symptoms include;

- ✓ Sensitivity to light from the sun or other sources.
- ✓ Seizures.
- ✓ Mouth or nose sores.
- ✓ Cold or stress-related pale or purple fingers or toes.
- ✓ Painful joints
- ✓ Eczema on the body
- ✓ Between the ages of 14 and 45, women are more likely than men to get lupus.
- ✓ Ankle enlargement.
- ✓ Pain in the chest while inhaling deeply.
- ✓ A malar rash is a butterfly-shaped rash that appears on the cheekbones and nose.
- ✓ Hair loss.
- ✓ Inflamed joints (arthritis).
- ✓ Consistent tiredness.

Systemic Lupus Erythematosus (SLE), Cutaneous Lupus (CL), Drug-Induced Lupus (DIL), and Neonatal Lupus (NL) (which affects infants whose mothers have SLE) are the several types of lupus. SLE occurs more frequently than the other types.

According to research, a 46-year-old woman with systemic lupus erythematosus received three intravenous doses of DMSO per month.

A 50% DMSO solution was injected and kept in place for an hour. Improvement was noted after each installation, and by the third treatment, no symptoms were present.

Also, a 31-year-old lady with systemic lupus erythematosus received 50 cubic centimeters (cc) of a 50% DMSO solution, which she was instructed to hold in her bladder for an hour on a monthly basis for three years. As a result, the symptoms subsided.

A

CHAPTER 21.

DMSO RECIPE AND APPLICATION FOR FUNGUS INFECTION TREATMENT.

DMSO is frequently used as a solvent for antifungal medications and fluconazole, an over-the-counter drug that works better to eliminate fungus when mixed with DMSO.

It has been established through numerous studies that DMSO has an inhibiting effect on the growth of dermatophyte colonies. Additional research was conducted to examine the impact of DMSO concentrations ranging from 0.125% to 10% on the development of fungus.

At 10% DMSO, there was no fungal growth, between about 2.5% and 7.5%, there was a linear dose inhibitory effect, and below 1%, there was a variable effect.

Lower DMSO concentrations that do not inhibit fungus growth may boost the effects of antifungal medications.

DMSO has been used to combine medications for the treatment of toenail fungus. Although DMSO does not directly affect the fungus, it functions as a driving force to aid other components in penetrating hard surfaces like nails.

It functions as a major enabler of other components and antifungals to immediately enter the fungus and eliminate it in its early stages.

A similar fungus infection known as athletes' foot has been successfully treated with DMSO, using concentrations of the compound ranging from 50% to 90% alone or in combination with capsicum and Aloe-vera.

By topically applying DMSO to the region of infection typically twice daily until the infection stops.

<u>DMSO RECIPE AND APPLICATION FOR INFLAMMATION TREATMENT.</u>

The body's immunological reaction to an irritant or foreign item is the inflammatory cycle. Inflammatory mediators such as histamine are released by the body's immune system, which causes the small blood vessels of the afflicted tissue to widen. This increases blood flow to the injured tissue, which causes the inflamed tissue to swell, the color red, and feel hot.

As an effective anti-inflammatory, DMSO lessens all signs and symptoms of inflammation. The body's anti-inflammatory hormone, cortisol, which is produced in the adrenal gland, is also more effective when combined with DMSO. When the body's cortisol concentration is low, it is still effective.

Non-Steroid Anti-Inflammatory Medicines, have adverse effects that are comparable to those of steroids, such as toxicity to the intestines and stomach, which can lead to pain, bleeding, and other problems. DMSO aids in the treatment of these adverse effects.

Due to its ability to scavenge free radicals, DMSO lessens gastritis caused by NSAIDs and aids in the repair of the digestive system.

DMSO has been used successfully in conjunction with diet and exercise to treat the majority of individuals with inflammations brought on by injuries and rheumatoid arthritis.

CHAPTER 22.

DMSO AND MIND HEALTH.

Disorders that impact thought, mood, and behavior are classified as mental health issues. When a mental health problem causes stress and interferes with daily activities or living, it is considered to be a mental disease.

DMSO has been used to treat a number of people with severe mental conditions such as schizophrenia, alcoholic psychosis, and severe anxiety.

A study was conducted on (forty-two) 42 patients in New York City, the patients were given DMSO in 5ml injections twice or three times daily at concentrations of 50% to 80% after entirely stopping all other drugs for roughly a week before treatment.

It was found that DMSO works better for addressing mental health issues in acute patients than in chronic ones.

<u>THE USE OF DMSO TO TREAT SKIN PROBLEMS.</u>

The majority of skin issues, including diabetic sores, infected wounds, and burns, respond well to DMSO treatment, according to a study conducted in Chile, individuals who had chronic skin ulcers that had been unsuccessfully treated with other treatments.

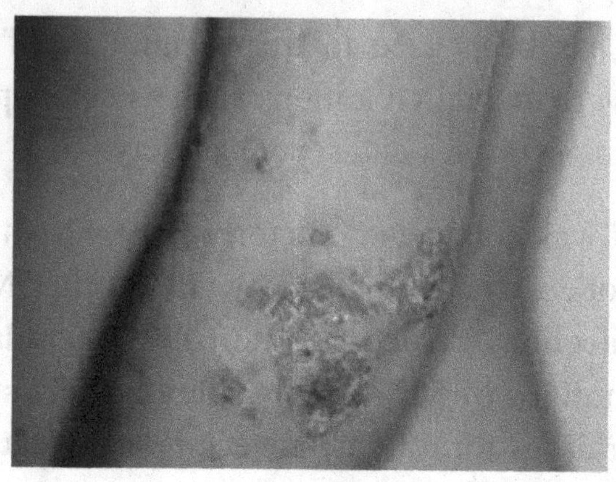

Three times a week, DMSO, antibiotics, and anti-inflammatory medications were used as the treatment. In situations with severe wounds, patients had some discomfort, but it did not interfere with the course of treatment and lasted only a short time. While some patients finished their treatments right away, others had to continue for a longer period.

An elderly man who had a two-inch-diameter ulcer brought about by damage to his varicose vein for over 15yrs was administered DMSO treatment. Although he had previously received therapy with different medications, the ulcer and sore were fully healed after nineteen (19) applications of DMSO spray.

CHAPTER 23.

RECIPE AND APPLICATION FOR TREATMENT OF MULTIPLE SCLEROSIS.

The Disease Multiple Sclerosis is a condition that affects the brain and spinal cord or the central nervous system. It causes the immune system to attack the myelin that protects nerve fibers, which interferes with body-to-brain communication and may cause irreversible nerve damage. Victims with multiple sclerosis may experience difficulty walking.

All ages are affected by multiple sclerosis, however, it is more common in women between the ages of 20-yrs and 40-yrs.

Thirty-four (34) patients with multiple sclerosis participated in an experiment with DMSO. The medication was discovered to be efficient and had a favorable impact on immunity, functions as an anti-allergic, and heals damaged tissue.

Patients with less severe conditions recovered quickly, but those whose conditions were fast progressing had unstable improvement with no adverse effects.

<u>SPINAL CORD INJURIES DMSO APPLICATION AND RECIPE.</u>

A major physical trauma that affects the spinal cord is called a spinal cord injury. We can move our limbs because of the spinal cord's role as a conduit for information between the brain and body.

Sensation and movement below the injured area are completely lost as a result of spinal cord damage. Arms and legs are affected by neck trauma (quadriplegia paralysis). It only affects the legs if it paralyzes the lower back region (paraplegia).

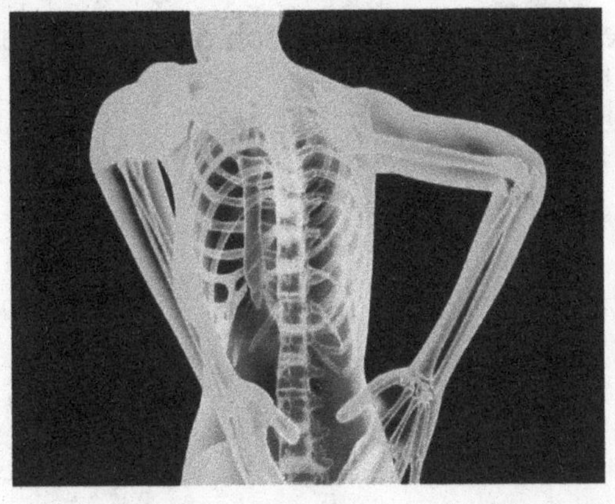

DMSO is a potent free radical scavenger that reduces swelling, boosts blood flow to injured areas, and increases oxygen availability at the spinal cord injury site.

Treatment with DMSO for spinal cord injuries can be administered intravenously using oral ingestion with juice or water, or locally on the affected area. DMSO should be provided as soon as the injury is sustained because it loses its effectiveness for permanent instances the longer it is left untreated.

After a severe spinal cord injury from a car accident, a man was able to move some body parts but was unable to walk, after administering DMSO lotion to his entire back three times each day for three months.

CHAPTER 24.

DMSO APPLICATION AND RECIPIENT INFORMATION FOR HERPES AND SHINGLES TREATMENT.

The varicella-zoster virus, which causes shingles, can infect any part of the body. However, it typically manifests as a band of blisters that wraps around the sides of the torso.

It develops years after chickenpox, lies dormant in the nerve tissue adjacent to the spinal cord and brain, and reactivates as shingles. The virus that causes this infection is the same virus that causes chickenpox.

Early intervention can minimize shingles infection and prevent consequences. Some of the shingles symptoms are;

- ✓ A few days after the pain, a red rash appears.
- ✓ Headache.
- ✓ Light sensitivity.
- ✓ Fatigue.
- ✓ Fluid-filled blisters that rupture and develop a crust.
- ✓ Itching.
- ✓ Fever.
- ✓ Numbness, tingling, burning, or pain.
- ✓ Touch sensitivity.

Typically, discomfort is the initial sign of shingles; but, occasionally, a rash will appear on the face, neck, or eyes.

Quadriplegia, or the paralysis of the arms and legs, can result from injuries to the top portions of the spinal cord in the neck. Lower back spinal cord injuries only result in paraplegia or paralysis of both legs.

HERPES:

Herpes is an illness that causes sores or blisters around the mouth or genitalia, as well as tingling, stinging, or burning.

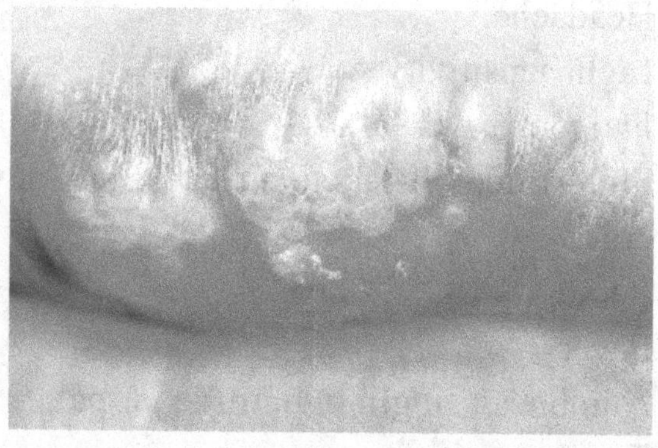

Herpes virus and other viral infections can be effectively treated with DMSO. When used early on,

DMSO is more effective in the treatment of shingles because it helps to reduce post-therapeutic neuralgia.

DMSO may be injected, taken orally, or directly administered to the afflicted area. According to a research on forty-three (43) patients, applying 50%–90% dimethylsulfoxide (DMSO) alone or with dexamethasone on the skin lesions, the patients recovered, with early treatment yielding the best outcomes.

A dermatologist in Argentina utilized a DMSO spray to treat patients with herpes zoster and herpes complicated. The patients responded well to the treatment when the spray was applied twice daily.

CHAPTER 25

DMSO APPLICATION AND RECIPE FOR DOGS AND HORSES, CHAPTER FIVE.

DMSO penetrates the skin to the blood in about 15-minutes in rats and about 60-minutes in dogs and horses when administered to the skin of rats, horses, and dogs.

According to research, a 15% DMSO was injected into the urinary bladder of sedated dogs to improve absorption. The procedure was then repeated to transport insulin via the bladder, and a decrease in blood sugar levels was seen.

It was also shown that certain substances, including steroids, vasoconstrictors, dyes, and skin antiseptics, can be absorbed via the skin of humans using both in-vivo and in-vitro methods.

The pharmacological effects of various medications were observed based on the behavior of the mice after their tails were dipped in a 5% DMSO and psychoactive solution. Water and other solvents were employed, and it was found that they penetrated.

It was shown that there were no anomalies after giving topical DMSO to four healthy dogs five days a week for 18 months at a rate of 1gram per kg of body weight.

DMSO solution should be applied directly to the skin on the affected area to treat acute edema caused by trauma.

When administering the medication to dogs with long hair, the hair is trimmed for simple drug monitoring. For Fourteen (14) days, 20ml of DMSO is administered twice or three times per day.

For 30 days, horses receive 100ml of DMSO twice or three times per day.

It is not suggested to use DMSO solution on dogs or horses who have an eye disease, liver or renal issues, allergies, or pregnancy. Dogs under 10-pounds, should not be administered DMSO.

For dogs, the daily maximum DMSO dosage shouldn't exceed 20-millimeters, and for horses, it shouldn't exceed 100-millimeters.

For both horses and dogs, the therapy period shouldn't exceed thirty (30) and fourteen (14) days, respectively.

DMSO should only be administered topically to animals, including horses and dogs. Under no circumstances may DMSO be given to horses that have been prepped for food or slaughter. A doctor should be consulted if any unfavorable effects of DMSO use are noticed.

CHAPTER 26
LASTLY.

Due to its therapeutic qualities, DMSO is respected as a significant product all over the world. There have been no reported reports of fatalities due to its use; it is used either alone or in combination with other products to treat a wide range of diseases.

Every clinician ought to be well-versed in DMSO and how it is used in clinical settings. DMSO can be used in cases with symptoms where the doctors are unable to reach a conclusion.

It is frequently disregarded by doctors who do not recognize or think that it can treat a wide variety of health issues. Because DMSO did not follow the accepted therapy recommendations as of then, researchers and physicians who examined and used it were attacked.

When DMSO is correctly used and controlled, organizations and the government spend less on healthcare, and people all over the world enjoy better, happier lives for less money.